I0436830

HOW
I Lost
Twenty Pounds

N Kept It Off

HOW
I Lost
Twenty Pounds

N Kept It Off

An Inspirational Tale of
Serendipity and Weight Loss

Caren Wong

Outskirts Press, Inc.
Denver, Colorado

The opinions expressed in this manuscript are solely the opinions of the author and do not represent the opinions or thoughts of the publisher. The author has represented and warranted full ownership and/or legal right to publish all the materials in this book.

How I Lost Twenty Pounds N Kept It Off
An Inspirational Tale of Serendipity and Weight Loss
All Rights Reserved.
Copyright © 2009 Caren Wong
v5.0

Cover Photo © 2009 JupiterImages Corporation. All rights reserved - used with permission.

This book may not be reproduced, transmitted, or stored in whole or in part by any means, including graphic, electronic, or mechanical without the express written consent of the publisher except in the case of brief quotations embodied in critical articles and reviews.

Outskirts Press, Inc.
http://www.outskirtspress.com

ISBN: 978-1-4327-4199-0

Outskirts Press and the "OP" logo are trademarks belonging to Outskirts Press, Inc.

PRINTED IN THE UNITED STATES OF AMERICA

Copyright Notice

Copyright 2009 By Caren Wong

All Rights Reserved. No part of this publication may be reproduced, stored in any retrieval system, transmitted in any form and by any means electronic, mechanical, photocopying, recording or otherwise without the prior written permission of the writer.

Legal Disclaimer

The writer at no point in this book claims to be a weight loss expert, nor does the writer guarantee the accuracy of all information contained herein. All experiences shared in this book are meant to be inspirational and not instructional. Please check with your physician when in doubt regarding whether any of the techniques for weight loss described herein are suitable for you. When in doubt, err on the side of caution or take responsibility for your own act of faith. The writer shall not be liable for any damages, ill health, or personal injuries resulting from following in her footsteps.

Author's Note

This book is dedicated to all you hundreds, thousands, or maybe hundreds of thousands of people out there who think you are "fat". Within these pages is a tale of my self-discovery and developing awareness of how my body works, what it needs and what it doesn't need. What foods am I sensitive to? To what extent can I cheat on my eating plans and still get away with it? Which foods make me gain weight and which help me lose weight? This book is also about my lost battles and ultimate victories throughout two decades of my life in relation to weight maintenance, and about how, I, as a human who loves to eat, finally developed a healthy relationship with food. I hope that reading about me will help you identify similarities in yourself, to strengthen your willpower and enable you to make wise decisions about your eating habits, bringing about the optimal weight you so desire. It is my wish that this story of mine will catalyze your own self-discovery and help you feel motivated, inspired, and encouraged in your fight against pudginess. Although we may be physically, metabolically, and genetically different, many of the food facts and rules of discipline and principles of healthy living I've discovered are universal. As a teenager growing up, I was often called "fat". The pain and anguish associated with being called thus caused me to set my life goal to be slim for as long as I live. May you find enlightenment, joy, discipline, and health in your journey towards your weight goals. Happy reading!

Acknowledgements

To my teachers in life for the past two years, Harv Eker and Robert G. Allen, who taught me the importance of using our talents, fanning our passions, and giving back to society.

Thanks to all who have called me "fat" because without you, I could still be fat and would not have given my life to discovering ways to losing weight and keeping it off!

To all the nutrition and weight-loss writers and journalists, who have shaped my beliefs and taught me so much about nutrition and weight loss. Special thanks to the coordinators, teaching and examining staff of GIFAM (Global Institute For Alternative Medicine) BSc in Holistic Nutrition course, for their wonderful inclusion of the important topic of Weight Loss in their curriculum.

Thanks to my sis, Brenna, and my friend, Joel Er, who have constantly asked me: "How is your book going?" Well, I am finally happy to say: It is in my hand and yours!

To my great fan and friend, Abdul Lathiff, who thinks so highly of me and ever believes in me.

To Rachit Dayal, Anthony John, Bo (aka Milton Periera) and Lathiff for all your timely endorsements.

Also, thanks to all you readers. This book is for you and because of you.

Endorsements

"This is a must read book for anyone on our streets trying to manage weight loss and still finding it hard to keep up the discipline.

Caren is my friend and client, and we the readers will be able to identify ourselves with her fight to make the impossible happen. Through her book she empowers each and everyone to make it happen, and weight loss will be your achievement if you and I can face it as Caren did.

It's a book that not only gives us tips on weight loss but a book that also gives us the confidence in our journey."

—Anthony John
Personal Trainer and Fitness coach

"Seems to be a common challenge among many of us. Weight Loss.

If you need to be assured that others are just like you, this is a perfect read. Caren manages to integrate a whole life's experience to show you that it is possible.

Whoever thought that walking can be such a miracle. Learn about having fun while doing it too. We as Singaporeans can identify the experiences of Caren, such as carrot cake, chendol, and ice kachang. I find the local flavor very adaptable with what us locals go through.

With more than a decade in the health and nutrition line and education, she was able to inculcate the right advice for the specific problem. The reader will garner many gems here.

You'll also find an excellent mix of biography on Caren's life journey and factual education on weight loss all at the same time. In other words, you'll feel as though the author is your long-time friend, and a smart one at that.

The Q & A section is also very refreshing and would be like taking advice from a friend.

Having known Caren for some time now, I must say that she has maintained her figure very well. So her words have certainly been put to action.

Live well and learn from the Caren's experience so you can avoid what not to do."

—Abdul Lathiff Jabar

"An excellent book that any layman can understand, finally! Caren has created a book with excellent observations on how to shed weight and maintain it. She has applied due diligence in self-study, done a little research, and has highlighted for us everyday things we can do that will be conducive to weight maintenance. And, if I were to change the title of the book, it would be "How to Lose Weight for Dummies! ... Kudos Caren!"

—Milton Pereira

"When Caren first sent over "How to Lose 20 Pounds N Keep It Off!!", I wasn't sure what to expect. I thought maybe it would be another generic weight loss book with the same old advice.

Boy, was I wrong! Caren's story of how she lost and kept off her excess weight is an inspiring story of lifelong learning and learning the art of self-discipline.

The book couldn't be more fun to read, and the advice is distilled and effective. I've also spent many years looking for the secrets of digestive health, and I completely agree with the diet and lifestyle principles she's discovered.

This is a book for anyone who has been watching their weight, their life, and wondering how other people manage to win their battles, and I whole-heartedly endorse the book. Excellent job, Caren!"

—Rachit Dayal
(Author of "*Secrets Of Irritable Bowel Relief*")

Table of Contents

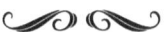

Introduction

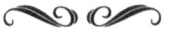

1

Introduction

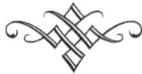

What follows is a story that spans two decades of how I lost **20 pounds** and kept it off. Once, I was overweight at 105 pounds, which was the highest I ever got! Friends called me "fat" then. Now my weight fluctuates between 85 to 87 pounds, and has remained thus since the year 2000, with a few slip-ups here and there. During these 20 years, I had my ups and downs. My techniques for weight control were pretty much trial and error. Some have been written about by other authors while some have not. The important thing was that each time I did something wrong, I took note of it, and when I recovered (meaning when I got to my ideal weight again), I "sinned" no more! There will be "fat" times and "thin" times throughout my story, and it was not until the year 2003 and after that I managed to stabilize my weight to the degree where I could say: I have got it! Throughout my journey, I also took risks about my body and questioned what I had been brought up to believe about food and made my own decisions. You can too!

I Wasn't Always Fat:

How did I grow up? How was I as a child? How did I eat? Well, as a 60's baby, I was fed off milk formulas. And during my growing up years till age 14, any discrimination of food between fat and thin, good and bad, healthy and unhealthy, was non-existent. Simply stated, I ate whatever my parents cooked, brought home, put on the table, or ordered at a restaurant. I remember that at age 11, I was eating three pieces of Kentucky Fried Chicken for dinner and did not feel any compunction. I remember also that at age seven, I could eat as many fish balls as I could stomach, and that was definitely more than three – giant ones. In fact, there was always some unseen competition between my cousins, siblings, parents' friends' children (when we visited or when they visited us) and I to see who could eat the most! It's silly when I think of it now because that could ruin our health, but back then, that was just the way it was! Furthermore, most adults I encountered at that time seemed to think that it was all right for us kids to eat as much as we wanted because we were still growing. How untrue! But at that time, I didn't know better. Well, it was with this kind of philosophy that my weight yo-yoed up and down, as I could see from the photos taken of me. In times of abundance, I was round, and in times of scarcity, I was trim, and I would say even attractive! But of course, that is in retrospect... Remember — I had no consciousness of these things as a child... My parents, for one, did not think being plump mattered, but on the contrary, my dad always told me to eat more when I got thin. So there I was, in a "plump trap", if you like. To my parents there was no fat and ugly. Just plump and cute, I guess. Some of you might disagree. I do now!

There are Proteins, Carbohydrates & Fats

My turning point came at age 15 when I was introduced to food facts in biology class. And what a revelation! I found myself absorbing, like a sponge, knowledge about proteins, carbohydrates and fats, as well as about the human digestive system. I seemed to have an aptitude for all this, and before long, biology became my second favorite subject (my favorite having been physical geography). One gram of protein yields four calories, as does one gram of carbohydrate, while one gram of fat yields nine calories. As for water, it has zero calories, and fiber is not only great for the bowels but you can also eat a kilo of it and still get very few calories! Based on my mistaken perception that all fats and oils were bad for the health and would make me fat[1] because it was high in calories, I launched into a campaign to avoid fats in all my meals. If the pork chop was fried in oil, I would dip it in my soup before eating it. Little did I know that sugars and carbohydrates are worse culprits when it comes to gaining weight.[2] So there I was, being fat free. The result of this campaign was that I became very thin, to the region of 79 pounds. My height is 1.55 m, so that meant my BMI was 14.9 (where the normal range is 18 to 22.9). My family even thought I was anorexic. In retrospect, maybe I was. Yet, it was none for the worse and not for long. I should consider myself lucky because all I did was err on the side of under-eating. There was nothing methodical about my weight loss till maybe the year 2000 onwards when

INTRODUCTION

I had more information. The things I thought were right, I just kept doing. There was nothing precise about the way I ate. I just ate fewer calories and kept my activity level high. I jogged, cycled, jumped rope, walked, and swam (swimming was my extra-curricular activity for six years in upper secondary and pre-university). Whenever I felt I had overeaten, I would simply "get rid of the calories" through exercise! All this while, my sister and grandmother nagged at me to put on weight but I ignored them. My satisfaction was more important. I was thin in Secondary Three, a little more fleshy in Secondary Four, and then I was thin throughout Pre-University I and II. All by trial and error, avoiding fats, and eating little!

How I Got Overweight

And so it came to pass that I went to the university ... Adapting to a new lifestyle and being in a course, LL.B (Honors), that I did not like dampened my spirits. In addition, five things stood out here, which I think led to my gaining weight to 105 pounds. If you remember, in my pre-university days, I was only around 79 pounds ...

- I had a hormone imbalance (or think that

was it) that caused my appetite to go out of whack.

- I developed irritable bowel syndrome[3] (IBS), which gave me irresistible urges to eat more.
- There were good cooked food stalls in the university that enticed me and caused me to compromise my strict rules of eating, amounting to loads of refined carbohydrates[4] with very little fiber.
- I snacked continually while I studied during my first and second year exams and stopped regular exercise.
- And of course, I dropped my fat-free ideology because fat was found in all the delicious fried food I found at the canteen. There was cooking oil in everything. It was as if nobody knew that cooking oil wasn't good for health! This misinformation and lack of information still exists to this day.[5]

One must wonder why after maintaining my weight at 79 pounds for three to four years, that I would suddenly give up my fight and surrender to my circumstances. The simple answer was that those urges to eat created by the hormonal

INTRODUCTION

imbalance and IBS, were so powerful as to render me totally helpless against them! Moreover, the negative stress I faced of having to excel in a course of study I had no aptitude for, made me depressed, unresourceful and lose my will power to stand up to temptation. All in all, I made pretty bad decisions that caused my weight to spiral up. At my heaviest, I was 105 pounds and became noticeably fat! One of my church mates, as well as pre-university classmate for two years, Clarence, took it so badly he had to tell me, "Hey! You have put on weight!" To which I replied, "Yeah!" And he said, "What do you mean yeah!?" Well, I guess his implication was that I should do something about it! Which I did.

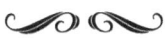

My First Step
To Recovery

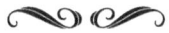

2

My First Step To Recovery

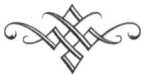

I Weighed Myself Every Day

The first thing I did was to buy a weighing scale. From that time on, I weighed myself every single day with no exception. I was 21 then.

I know what you are going to say: You read somewhere that someone or some expert said one should not weigh oneself every day? But why not? Weighing daily nips the damage in the bud. It puts us on guard and tells us if what we chose to eat that day was gaining or losing us weight. But please note the following guidelines for daily weighing that I set for myself:

- I weighed myself every morning because that was when I am lightest, which made me feel encouraged.

- I did not panic when I weighed myself at night and found I gained three pounds. This weight gain included the food and fluids I consumed that day.
- My clothes were a secondary corroboration to whether I had gained weight.

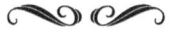

From 105 to 95 (1986)

3

From 105 to 95 (1986)

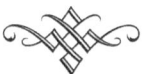

I Discovered Walking

This is the greatest miracle in my weight loss story so far. I was in university then, and after I failed my second year of law school, I decided to rent a room near campus in order to save time on traveling, which meant I would have more time for reading and revision – every undergraduate's dream. This place was at West Coast (near Clementi). At that time, my regular exercise was still swimming. Then, one fortuitous night, about a month after I moved in, I decided to go for a walk around the estate. As I loved nature, I veered towards the remote seaside, open fields and less traveled highway, away from the blocks of HDB (Housing and Development Board) flats. It was a quite a long walk, about half an hour. But because the sea breeze and solitude were so delightful, I decided to walk again the following night—and the night after the following night, and so forth, until it became a habit. This habit turned out to be my lifesaver. Within one week, my weight dropped from 105 to 95 with no change in my sleeping habits or the amount of food I ate[6], which was already little. The first question I asked myself was: what was I doing different that could have caused this phenomenal change? The answer was undoubtedly my nightly walk. Because of my faith that walking was then a much better form of exercise for me, I dropped swimming. After all, if swimming didn't do it for me that one month before this "miracle", then it wouldn't work even if I continued. I mean, I wasn't gaining weight through swimming, but then again, I wasn't losing weight either. Other benefits I experienced after I started walking were mental alertness and improved self-esteem, which were so precious to me at that time because of the stigma of having to repeat my second year of university.

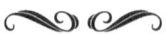

From 95 to 92 (1988)

4

From 95 to 92 (1988)

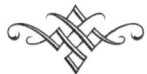

My First Years Working

Okay, so I continued on as a student through the third and fourth year. Right up till graduation, I remained at 95 pounds. After graduating, I bummed around for a while and rented a room at Towner Road. Goodness knows how I survived, but survive I did. My meals were scanty, so putting on weight was never an issue.[7] After a while, my father caught up with me and insisted I join a law firm to do a pupilage. He called my cousin, Wong Chak Wing (still a practising lawyer), who then called his friend, Peter Chua of the then "Peter Chua, Sobaran and Partners", to take me on as pupil. Peter agreed. So there I was, a pupil at a law firm. It was here at the law firm that I got used to wearing office clothing—the straight skirt, the long sleeved silky blouse, and the empowering dark jacket—all very professional. This change in wardrobe proved a bonus to me in my lifelong goal to never be fat again. How so? Well, in order to get into the same non-stretchable skirt every day, I had to eat the same certain amount of food daily. Now, this wasn't easy, for as everyone can well relate to, foods are never served with a piece of paper telling you how many calories they have to start with, or that if you left behind a slice of meat or a spoonful of rice, then you will be ingesting x number of calories less! So I had to exercise extreme caution, as well as keen observation of my body's response towards whatever I consumed. For example, if I ate spinach with a tablespoon of rice and some tofu at lunch, that would still leave room for me to eat a dinner of home-cooked kangkong, chicken drumstick, and sandwich slice without putting on weight. That would add up to about 800 calories a day max! Too little? Well, for my size and body weight, it was about right, as I was later to discover in August 1998 when I read an article in Let's Live magazine.[8] Here, Mr Bill Carpenter MS, RD shared that there is a calorie formula for losing, maintaining, and gaining weight based on our target weight.

This is summarized in the table below:

	No. of Calories consumed per day	With Moderate Activity/Exercise
To Lose Weight	Target Weight in Pounds x 8	X 1.5
To Maintain Weight	Target Weight in Pounds x 10	X 1.5
To Gain Weight	Target Weight in Pounds x 12	X 1.5

So for me, if I wished to maintain my weight at 85 pounds, I would have to take in only 850 calories without exercise, and about 1270 calories with moderate activity or exercise — astonishingly little compared to what most people eat!

In case anyone should forget, all this while, walking was still my exercise. It was a blessing that I could walk away my weight in case I made any mistakes and felt the gain in my waistline, which occurred every so often. For example, if instead of eating a proper vegetable-based lunch, I chose to eat a medium-sized coconut tart with a medium-sized deep fried curry puff, not only would I experience less efficient bowel movements, I would also feel the gain in my waist. It was my sensitivities that kept me on the narrow path.

HOW I LOST TWENTY POUNDS...

My First Pitfall After Graduation

Not long after, I had to interrupt my pupilage to attend a postgraduate Practical Law Course (PLC) together with 100 others, conducted by the Adult Legal Education Board. The PLC was a prerequisite to being admitted to the bar, which of course was what my father wanted for me. It was there at the PLC that I started gaining weight again, much to my chagrin. Once again, the cause was uncontrolled eating. I couldn't believe it was happening again. What seemed to be a perfect figure was ruined after just days of eating the wrong foods again (which at that time, I did not have the savvy to classify as such). I remember the ice kachang[9] and "chai tow kueh" (stir-fried carrot cake) I ate at People's Park Hawker Center every day. Luckily for me, the course ended before my weight gain became too disastrous to manage or lose. I went back to Peter Chua to finish the remaining days of my pupilage. During that time, I took the chance to lose the weight I had gained through walking from a bus stop (two stops away) to my office at Beach Road. I also went back to my usual vegetable meals, but my weight was a constant 95 pounds and did not get below 90. Subconsciously, I was aiming for my pre-university weight of 79 pounds. And never have I eaten fried carrot cake together with ice kachang[9] at one sitting since.

Helped by a Centipede Bite

At the time of my pupilage, my parents and I stayed in a terrace house in Soo Chow Gardens. It was a civilized place with cement compound and mosaic flooring in the kitchen, not the kind of place you would expect to find creepy crawlies. But, one of them did appear. It was a giant-sized centipede that was broad and brownish yellow in color, which according to experts, was considered "old" and would have bitten many a person. Guess where it appeared? On our fridge door!! What happened was when I opened the fridge to get a snack (how ironical), this giant centipede was already hovering at the base of the fridge door. So, when I opened the door, the creature conveniently slithered onto my right foot and bit my right big toe. I could see the puncture marks instantly, and started to feel an excruciating pain that came in throbs and surges. My right leg began to swell, and by the time I reached the Toa Payoh Hospital Accident and Emergency Department (now defunct), the swelling had reached my right knee. My right leg was enormous and the degree of pain I felt was beyond anything I had ever experienced. Usually a quiet girl, I had an instant change of personality as a result of the pain. I talked non-stop and yelled for attention until a nurse on duty gave me priority and attended to me. They injected me with a dose of morphine and wheeled me to a hospital bed where I was to spend the night. Two hours on, I was still crying in pain and talking non-stop. The nurse had to inject me again and again. In total, I had three morphine injections. One of the nurses who attended to me later told me that I was very strong. Normally, a person would have been knocked unconscious with the dosages administered to me. At that time, I didn't question what stopped the swelling or the progression of the poison. I was just happy to be alive.

I was discharged the following evening after having made one friend (the girl on the next bed). The minute I reached home, I went for my jaunt around the estate. I had lost my appetite totally. I guess I was still recovering from the shock. However, I was sane enough to weigh myself. The scales registered 92 pounds! Finally, a drop in weight. And just by not eating for 24 hours!

FROM 95 TO 92 (1988)

Good job!

The moral of this story is that we may eat or snack out of habit, without realizing that an interruption of this habit may actually be good for us and our weight. In my case, my encounter with that centipede bite and hospital stay interrupted my eating, and because of that, I dropped three pounds. Effectively, that was involuntary fasting for a day. The consequence of dropping three pounds was that I felt a great sense of satisfaction. This further meant that any time I wished, I could voluntarily fast for one day and drop three pounds. That would not be impossible but it would take willpower, something I didn't usually have, because like everybody else, I love to eat! So you could say, I was helped by a centipede bite.

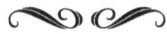

From 92 to 86 (1989)

5

From 92 to 86 (1989)

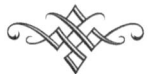

My Stint at Cane Creations

After my pupilage was over, I hunted around for a job. After a few temporary positions, I ended up in a furniture shop called Cane Creations (now defunct) as a retail assistant. This company was started by a shipping magnate as a sideline. During this time, I learnt to read food labels. My working hours were either from 10 am to 6 pm or from 12 pm to 9 pm, so that gave me plenty of free time. To unwind from my job, I would visit 7-eleven after work. One day, on a whim, I read that a slice of Sunshine bread was 75 calories. Suddenly, it dawned upon me that I could continue to learn the calorie value of food items just by continuing to read labels. In other words, I didn't have to pay to learn. I considered this another turning point. Knowledge would be potential power. This could turn out to be useful in due time. So whenever I came upon some information, I would memorize the figures. I was slowly picking up. Every now and then I would learn something new about calories, food, and weight. Looking back, I think my whole life was meant to be a lesson unto myself so I could teach others. Why then was I so interested and passionate about it? While others would just go out and buy a new shirt, blouse, or skirt, I would insist on keeping my weight constant so I could fit into the same old clothes for a long time to come. That gave me a sense of accomplishment.

The second greatest event in this phase of my life was the changing of my working hours from rotating shifts to regular hours. What used to be 10 am - 6 pm, rotating with 1 pm - 9 pm, became 11 am - 7 pm every single day. As a result, I dropped 6 pounds to 86.

Self-Observation, Hypothesis Creation

Each time my weight dropped dramatically, I would put forth a hypothesis about myself. This time was no different. My hypothesis was that getting up later than usual and having fixed hours of work as opposed to shift work was conducive towards weight loss and weight maintenance. In other words, if I kept regular hours of work and sleep every day, it would be more helpful towards weight control than if I were to do irregular hours of work and sleep and get up at different times every day. Based on my self-observation, this hypothesis held true for me. As a result, I ate little. I guess this has something to do with my diurnal rhythm, which if I were in sync with, would lead to appetite control. In that way, I was helped towards my weight goals. I was definitely making progress and getting closer to my target of 79 pounds.

During this time, I also:

- Got used to eating 8 oz meals (around the size of a fist or slightly more). Working in a stress-free environment caused my appetite to drop. At times, I even felt I was force-feeding myself.

- Read a book or two during my free time about weight loss. One was "28 Day Metabolic Plan"[10] and the second was "Walk, Don't Die"[11]. These simply reinforced my learning and assured me that I was on the right track. My most important lesson from the first book was to eat everything with vegetables, for when we do, less of the oils and carbohydrates will enter our bloodstream. This helped me a lot towards maintaining my weight at 86 pounds.

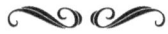

Staying At 86 (1990)

6

Staying At 86 (1990)

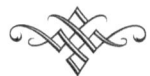

My Stint at Company X (flexi hours)

Soon after Cane Creations closed down, I joined a commodities trading company. The lifestyle here was a blast. My team and I woke up late, ate together a lot, and worked only a minimal of four hours a night. During our working hours, we were served Chinese tea. From here, I discovered that drinking tea keeps the waist small. What was also memorable this season of my life were:

- Waking up late meant I ended up eating less for that day. I realized then that working office hours meant one starts the first meal too early in the day. Higher calories would be consumed by the end of the day.
- My colleagues were very receptive to my

style of eating when I made it known. I had totally no issues with my teammates, who would continue to order their meals in large quantities (but smaller quantities for me). We got along just fine.

- I walked a lot during this season to and from office to the nearest bus stop, and this did me good.

My Stint as an Executive Assistant (Office)

My lifestyle here was a total opposite of the earlier company:

It was characterized by:

- Getting up early. Not my cup of tea, as for me it was associated with being out of sync and gaining weight.
- Being in the office by 9 am.
- Rigid hours of 9 am to 6 pm Mon-Fri, with Sat and Sun off.
- Eating rigidly at lunch time, which was either 12 noon or 1 pm whether I felt hungry or not.
- Snacking on sweets while working on the word processor.

STAYING AT 86 (1990)

Nothing disastrous happened to me here but I just felt there were many risks hovering around (especially the sweet habit while typing) that might prove detrimental to my long-term weight goals. After all, there was plenty of sitting down, not a good posture for maintaining weight, or so it occurred to me at that time. In addition, the rigid hours of eating were enough to take the enjoyment out of it. One should only eat when hungry, so I thought. And during a meeting, visiting the bathroom would be an issue even if I said: excuse me. So the bottom line was: office job? Not conducive for weight maintenance!

I continued to walk after work for exercise, and this continued to do me good. It was also during this time that I discovered the wonders of popiah.

Popiah[12] – A Slimming Food

One fine day, after being stressed out by typing and office work, and having the feeling that I had already exceeded my calorie intake for that day (because I had sweets while typing), I went to Chinatown for a walk. On the way home, I sat down for a freshly rolled popiah (not the deep-fried type), thinking that: this is it. I am going to gain a pound again. Drats! But no ... The next morning when I awoke, lo and behold, my waist was slim, slim, slim! By chance, I chose a food that satisfied my emptiness without blowing me up. Just what I needed. Either that or it was the popiah meal coupled with the long walk I had after that. The bottom line was: the more "thin factors" I put into practice, the faster I would reach my goals. So, what about popiah is slimming?

In a nutshell, it may look enormous, taste delicious and fill you up, but actually has few calories. Let's take a closer look why this is so.

First, it is made of 80% vegetables, three to be exact: turnip, bean sprouts, and green lettuce. And these, though they form the bulk of the *popiah*, are extremely low in calories(a little less than 100 probably). The other ingredients are just a little sliced and diced hardboiled egg, maybe some prawns and deep-fried shredded batter, which contribute to a few more tens of calories. Finally, there is garlic paste, chilli sauce, and dark sweet sauce, which are spread onto the popiah skin, which together carry the bulk of the calories in the entire dish. The turnip is stir-fried and stewed in gravy with some or a lot of oil depending on who prepares it. Usually, when the vendor scoops the turnip onto the popiah skin, he would squeeze it semi-dry so that the better part of the cooking oil is drained off. This really does save us some calories. If you are carbohydrate sensitive, simply leave out the skin and eat just the vegetables and other filling. But it'll do you no harm to eat the entire concoction (which tastes better) because the total calorie count would be just a little over 200 calories. That would be about a third of the usual "rice with dishes" meal. In order to save even more calories, you may request the one who prepares it for you not to include the deep-fried shredded batter and put less sweet sauce!

Another theory I derived from this was that if our last meal of the day were plain vegetables, our weight loss would be accelerated. I put this to the test later on and realized it was true. However, I seldom used this tactic because I prefer eating a balanced meal of vegetables, protein, and a little carbohydrate no matter what time of day I ate. Only on drastic occasions would I practice eating pure vegetables.

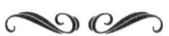

From 86 to 79 (1991)

7

From 86 to 79 (1991)

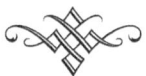

At Family Health Foods

After I decided I had enough of office work that was heading nowhere, I found Family Health Foods (now defunct), a retailer of health food and supplements. The first outlet I worked in was United Square. This turned out to be my long-term career – retailing in health and nutrition. Weight maintenance was just one part of the entire package. It was a perfect match. Within a month, I could tell I was made for this and I lamented that I had not found this earlier. Why so? Well:

- Our job required us to stand, which burned more calories than sitting.
- It required us to do price tagging and shifting things around when changing displays or

stacking goods (more calories expended).

- It required us to do housekeeping: sweep, mop, and clean shelves (more calories expended).

- It required us to talk and interact with people, which not only burned calories but kept our minds and adrenals stimulated.

- It required continual learning about our fascinating human body and related fields. It was as if I had come full circle since biology class in Secondary Three and continued my purpose in life – to find out as much about health and nutrition as possible and to be an example of how to beat stress, aging, weight gain, and illness.

Imagine what a head start I would have had, had I found this job earlier! But, as I had learned to always say: There is a time for everything; better late than never; everything happens for a reason; And no permanent damage.

Regular Working Hours

Knowing that getting up late and regular hours would be conducive towards maintaining a steady weight, I requested for a permanent afternoon shift, which was from 1 pm to 9 pm. The position involved a six-day week with one flexible day off a week. Imagine getting up at 11 am every morning, reaching my work place at 1 pm, and finishing punctually at 9 pm.... Life was a blast! On my days off, I went for long walks, mostly in shopping malls or Changi Airport, and ate as little as I could.

Being Nitpicky With Food

I realized that since my target weight, body size, and low metabolism would not permit me to eat with abandon, I had to choose my meals very carefully. A few rules were definitely in place already. **No doubling, no force-feeding, and most importantly, eat everything with soft, pulpy vegetables.** This requires a little explanation. No doubling means that when faced with a choice whether I should eat dish A or dish B to go with my rice, I would pick just one but not both because picking both would mean eating to discomfort and doubling my quota of calories for that meal. Every meal would have at least one serving of vegetable and one serving of protein. No force-feeding meant that if I had chosen a meal that was unpredictable and it turned out not to satisfy my gustatory standards, then I would just leave it and not eat it. If I forced myself, the food would not be well digested and I would continue to crave for an alternative. In all probability, I would stuff. This meant eating even when full.

I picked **soft, pulpy vegetables** because they were good for my bowels and because they gave me a perfect feeling of satiety unlike hard stringy ones.

In other words, all meals were chosen carefully, treated with respect, and enjoyed with no distractions, such as reading the papers or watching television. Every bit, every mouthful, every crunch would be savored with delight and sensuality. This works best in solitude. It's also such a luxury, and I didn't have to pay much for it. In fact, the most enjoyable good tastes may turn out to be the cheapest. I just had to know where to find them, or how to prepare them. Plus, **every meal had to have just the right proportion, which was 8 oz or "fist sized".** Please note that I did all these by trial and error and self-awareness. In the years that followed, some of my methods and theories were vindicated by some renowned researchers in the field of nutrition and weight maintenance.[13]

FROM 86 TO 79 (1991)

In my case, human experience preceded scientific knowledge. I had an experience that caused me to hypothesize, which then caused me to make further observations to either verify or invalidate that hypothesis. It helped greatly that others had done the research to corroborate my personal experiences. Truth is indeed universal and science is just reality waiting to be discovered.

Maslow's Theory

During working hours and in-between customers, I read ferociously. I was lucky that when I joined the company there were many health books in the inventory. So I took the liberty.

One of the authors that made a deep impression on me was Dr Maslow[14] (not the famous psychologist who came up with the Hierarchy of Needs Theory). He was a fruitarian nutritional doctor and experimented with bread until he died. But the point of his book was that the human digestive system goes through three phases: the resting phase, the elimination phase, and the feeding phase. The resting phase is from 9 pm right till 9 am. Elimination is between 9 am and 1 pm, which is why humans should only eat at

1 pm or after. And feeding time was 1 pm to 9 pm. When I read that, I thought to myself: No wonder I don't feel like eating in the morning. Later on, when I interviewed some people I came across, I realized that not everybody was like that. Some of my colleagues actually got up feeling hungry. For these people, not eating breakfast meant not being functional. How was I to reconcile Dr Maslow's theory, which I fitted neatly into, with what I observed in others? I couldn't. But that did not stop me from applying what I felt was relevant in my situation. So from then on, my first meal of the day was always after 12 noon. Occasionally, I did get hungry around 11:30 am, due to starting work earlier. When that happened, I did not deny myself. But mostly, I had my first meal late, which (you might have guessed) was 8 oz, fist-sized, or just slightly more.

Books Helped

Some of the other books in the store talked about our digestive system, intestinal cleansing, and fasting for health. I found them intriguing, especially photographs of impacted fecal matter. It was scary yet fascinating that we could store so much unwanted waste in our colon — a major cause of weight gain and other diseases. A pithy saying from Dr Maslow's book stayed with me. It was: "Better a day of controlled eating than to buy a day of feasting with the fast of many." Till now, this and many more axioms have stuck with me.

Definition of Constipation

But the bombshell was Patricia Bragg's book[15] on Apple Cider Vinegar. She mentioned that the natural bowel movements of humans should be once after every meal but that our modern lifestyle has changed our ability to respond to that natural rhythm, to our detriment. If we could only go back to that way, we would be healthier, with fewer incidences of colon cancer and other forms of illness. An unhealthy colon, according to her and other experts in this field, was the usual starting point for disease to take place. So to stay healthy, keep the bowels open. Better still, start fasting and cleansing your system on a regular basis.

In Bragg's opinion, if undigested food stays in our system for more than 24 hours, we are considered constipated. In other words, whatever you ate last night should be out by tonight. Such a strict standard left me awestruck! But I recovered and chose to accept and adopt it as my standard. From then on, I was very observant of my bowels. Naturally, this had a beneficial effect on weight maintenance. After all, regular bowel movements meant that there would be little chance for re-absorption of calories and toxins, and therefore, less accumulation of fats (fat, water, and toxins tend to agglutinate). My observations of myself led me to discover that hard meat slowed down my bowels (but not so much minced meat), and vegetables reduced transit time. As a result, I became a partial vegan who ate poultry or fish once in two weeks only and minced pork only say once in six months. I can't say for sure. But my frequency of eating hard meat definitely became small.

Calorie Counting Books

Other books I came across included calorie and fat counters written by western authors, which were not entirely relevant here in Singapore, but I gleaned and applied whatever information I could. Today, the Singapore Health Promotion Board (HPB) has a publication[16] that makes it much easier to size up the calorie value of some local food, making calorie counting a cinch.

Bout of Diarrhea

All went well at Family Health, United Square, in terms of weight control. In fact, after one bout of diarrhea, my weight dropped to 79 pounds. But the minute I started eating a little more, my weight went back up above 80. I had a hunch I was still growing (even though I was already 27 because I had a really late menarche), so I allowed it to happen. Although I wanted to be slim, I didn't want to be malnourished and emaciated either. I was spot on in terms of my goal, but keeping that 79 pounds was really painful, because the routine was unbearable. My calorie intake had to be somewhere between 600-800 calories, and no more, even with exercise. For me, that was hardly eating. And this allowed me no cheating or snacking, which I loved doing. You see, the lower you want your weight to be, the less you can eat. But I loved to eat and I was eating in the region of 1000 calories per day (with exercise) and that led me to hover between 83 and 85 pounds. It was then that I decided to throw in the towel and declare 83-85 to be my permanent weight target for my remaining sojourn on earth.

79 pounds was simply too punishing.

That Time of the Month

One large detail that kept recurring during this time was that every once in a while, for seemingly no reason, I felt bloated and fat even without binging or breaking any rules. It troubled me for a great many years. I was later to find out that this has something to do with women's hormonal cycles — progesterone and estrogen, to be more precise. Generally, progesterone is the slimming one and estrogen is the water and fat retentive one. This subject proves confusing even for someone with my background[17], and I am still reading up on it and attempting to understand it all. Be that as it may, my shallow understanding of this phenomenon was enough to put me on guard against those monthly ups and downs and the possibility of an accumulation of fat if I were to be careless in my eating. Shedding the gains could prove less than easy. One sure sign that progesterone is on the rise is when I can eat more than usual and still not put on weight. And here's the rub. A few days later, after I get so used to eating "a lot", not putting on weight and enjoying it, progesterone takes a dive, which will cause just the opposite effect! Whatever I eat seems to cling on to me or cling on inside me and any effort to lose it seems futile. So rule of thumb is: **Even when I think I can eat all I want and not put on weight, I don't.** This could be that time of the month when glory precedes misfortune.

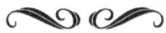

Staying Below 86
(1993-1996)

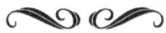

8

Staying Below 86 (1993-1996)

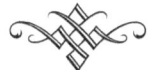

Bukit Timah Plaza

After two years at Family Health's outlet at United Square, I was transferred to Bukit Timah Plaza. Here, my healthy diet of home-cooked vegetable and 8 oz, fist-sized meals was interrupted by the convenience of eating Colonel Burger from Kentucky Fried Chicken, which was just a stone's throw from where I worked. It was the economy (just $1.70 each) and convenience of purchasing this burger that made me shelf the vegetable-based and 8 oz fist-sized routine. But most of all, it was the sheer delight of biting into the juicy, tasty, tender chicken patty that kept me on this menu for the full three months I was there. Anyway, this burger had not much calories, probably about 300 or less (if half of the bun was left uneaten). And that was about all I ate for the day. Despite that, my weight did not go down, perhaps because of the lower workload. Less customer traffic meant fewer calories expended. During this time, I had fun dating, another reason for the lowered appetite, I guess.

At Chinatown Point

After Bukit Timah, I was transferred to Chinatown Point. This marked the end of my permanent afternoon shift simply because my colleague, Katherine, requested that I rotate shifts with her. And so I did. By then, I already had an arsenal of tricks up my sleeve to stay thin despite the irregular hours, and continued to read labels and memorize calorie counts. Therefore, juggling my weight was not such a big deal, especially with walking as exercise.

Here is a sample list of the caloric values I already knew by that time:

1 slice of bread	75 calories
1 Big Mac	480 calories
6 pc McDonald's chicken nuggets	460 calories
1 small Mac Fries	260 calories

STAYING BELOW 86 (1993-1996)

1 bottle organic apple juice	80 calories
1 orange	90 calories
1 cup of coffee with sugar & cream	100 calories
1 decent rice meal with vegetables	6-700 calories

The biggest snag, however, was my appetite and food cravings. Imagine that if I had totally no appetite, then it would be impossible for me to overeat, wouldn't it? But this was not the case. In other words, I had to observe and learn ways to keep my appetite down. These were some things I discovered:

- I had to love what I was doing.
- I had to keep relatively busy.
- I had to have proper rest and recreation.
- I had to sleep well, as poor sleep led to cravings to eat throughout the following day.
- I had to eat foods in the right proportion and amount.
- I had to keep salt and sugar in food and drinks to a minimum and also snack as little as possible on chocolates and sweets.

When all else failed, I exercised sheer grit and self control plus erred on the side of under eating.

But life was not without its challenges and bloopers! One fine day, I decided to eat a dessert, called chendol[18]. This was full of coconut milk and *gula melaka* or palm sugar. The minute I finished, I felt it on my waist. My hypothesis: My body does not metabolize coconut milk and/or gula melaka (palm sugar) well. So it didn't matter that I did not eat it often and it didn't matter that I did not finish the entire bowl. As a result, that was the last chendol I had for many years to come.

At Suntec City

Not long after the chendol affair, our company opened a new outlet in Suntec City and I was asked to head it.

At Suntec City, I worked with a lady who loved to eat curry puffs from a café near our store. I decided to join in whenever she did eat, which was every other day. I also remembered that for the two short months I was at Suntec, I was eating Nestlé Lion bars on a regular basis. That must have contained at least 240 calories per bar! Despite this apparent unhealthy, non-weight-smart change in eating habit for me, I was fortunate not to go beyond 86 pounds. That didn't mean, however, that I was looking my best. Two other factors may have contributed to my limited weight gain. I ate only twice a day rather than three times (loss of appetite again, but this time, due to the open working environment), and also because my walk to and from the bus stop was about 10 minutes each, enough to burn off some calories.

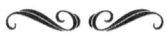

Fine-Tuning Years
(1997 to 1999)

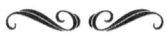

9

Fine-Tuning Years
(1997 to 1999)

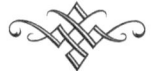

In Year 1997, I joined yet another health food chain, GNC. At that time, it was still a small company. My time here was quite an adventure (as I worked in more than seven different outlets throughout my first five to six years), and it was a period of personal growth as well as deepening knowledge in the field of nutrition, weight maintenance, and customer service. I continued to have many revelations, bloopers, and victories with regards to weight. These are too many to recall and document in a little book like this. So I shall only go for the salient, unforgettable ones.

Close-Fitting Clothes

The first thing that changed in 1997 was my

new uniform, which was a figure-hugging shift dress. In order to ensure I could wear it every day, I had to watch what I ate — not that I wasn't already watching. But I had to be extra careful, especially in the beginning. Outside of my working hours, my regular outfits varied throughout the years. But I kept it really consistent and tighter fitting so that I could tell when my waistline was expanding. Most of the people around me thought my clothes were my uniform. But no, that wasn't it, and it was also NOT that I was lazy to change my clothes. I just did not think wearing loose-fitting clothes was a good idea in my situation, as that would make me less wary of exceeding my boundaries.

Some other lessons, in a nutshell, during this period were:

- Air-conditioning and cold drinks stimulate fat burning.
- Deep-fried foods caused me weight gain.
- Protein and vegetables are a better choice than carbohydrate and vegetables (for me at any rate).
- Pastries with lard are a fast way to gain weight, e.g. BBQ pork pastry.

Ate More Than Two Hours Apart

During a very boring and non-peak season in 1998 at the United Square outlet, I had a relapse of uncontrolled eating. I ate every two hours. The pattern would be pineapple, papaya, and deep-fried curry puff spaced two hours apart. These were not even my normal diet. I only ate them because they were easily available from a coffee shop nearby and someone offered to buy them for me! These items were not fattening per se, but it was the timing plus my own body's low metabolism and low activity level. In other words, if another person with high metabolism ate the way I did, it would probably not cause him or her a gain in weight. After all, the total calorie count of what I ate was only about 500 calories. And if I added that to whatever else I ate that day, it would have been 1100 to 1200 calories — little by average standards. Whatever it was worth, I registered these lessons into my subconscious.

<u>Lesson One</u>: Be sure to eat more than two hours apart.

<u>Lesson Two</u>: Everything has calories, fruits included. i.e. It is possible to gain weight by eating pineapple and papaya IF they are in addition to what I usually eat. In retrospect, sugar in fruit may

contribute to even faster weight gain than a piece of whole grain bread.

Lesson Three: Low activity days should not serve as opportunities to eat more, but rather to put myself on guard to NOT eat as a filler. Finding something to do would have been more beneficial.

I should also mention that as a result of this setback, I could not wear my uniform comfortably, and this served to reinforce my conviction that letting go and throwing caution to the wind was not and would never be worth it no matter how enjoyable eating was. Short-term pleasure, long-term pain!

"The" Formula

One fine day, in the month of August 1998, I chanced upon an article that proved to be a turning point in my life. This article was in Let's Live Magazine[19], and the contributor was Bill Carpenter, M.S. R.D. He called his article the Lose/Gain Formula. Of course, you have already come across this under the chapter on my early years of working, but here, I've reproduced it for convenience.

At that time, I was already on a weight-loss

FINE-TUNING YEARS (1997 TO 1999)

	No. of Calories consumed per day	With Moderate Activity/Exercise
To Lose Weight	Target Weight in Pounds x 8	X 1.5
To Maintain Weight	Target Weight in Pounds x 10	X 1.5
To Gain Weight	Target Weight in Pounds x 12	X 1.5

path, after one bout of indulgence (my indulgences occurred from time to time). While I was struggling to get below 85, this formula not only blew me away but propelled me to such action that my weight went down to 79 pounds again. This got me so excited it gave me a high for days on end, plus so much confidence. It was as if my whole life was waiting for this moment to manifest itself! This truth certainly set me free and gave me plenty of answers. And in case anyone has any doubt as to its feasibility, the results I got by putting it to the test certainly removed any iota of doubt. How brilliant can these nutritional scientists get! From then on, I knew exactly how to get where I wanted by changing my calorie intake and taught others to do the same (if they would listen of course. Usually they don't, because the calorie intake suggested seemed ludicrously low compared to what they would usually eat). But I must admit, it took courage and determination to stand by the numbers and ignore my hunger pangs after I had eaten past that number. So if you want to follow this formula, be prepared to be very resolute! Caveat: the multiplier factor can be enhanced to 1.8 for very active people, as opposed to the just moderately active. If one is inactive, it would be best to stick with the factor of 8 for losing and 10 for maintaining.

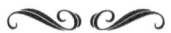

A Time of Ups and Downs (Year 2000)

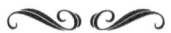

10

A Time of Ups and Downs (Year 2000)

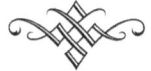

At Novena Square

In the year 2000, I was given yet another chance to head a new outlet, the one at Novena Square. This was a time when I faced many temptations, got into a sweet habit big time, as well as ate plenty of chocolates. All in all, my weight would yoyo from 82 to 87 and then back to 82 over six-month periods. At that time, I had a three-year-old nephew who also enjoyed candies, so keeping off candies was an issue as I had good company. It gave me a sense of satisfaction to be able to supply the candies without having to finish them all as I had him to share them with.

My second aberration was that I was influenced by my colleagues in some respects of food choices.

HOW I LOST TWENTY POUNDS...

Our cooked meals were purchased from the then Novena Square Food Court. Even though I did not eat that much, I did include at times into my menu, refined carbohydrates, which were not supposed to be in my diet. Examples include minced pork noodles and fried carrot cake, plus fried kuay teow, which I vowed never to eat back in my early years of working. There were also meat dishes that I would not usually eat, for instance, "sweet and sour chicken thigh" with the skin on. Again, this caused me to gain weight immediately, especially around the waist. As a result, I could not eat these consistently unlike my colleagues. (This dish has much hidden sugar in the vinegar sauce.) At the Novena Square Food Court, there was also a Malay stall selling my favorite vegetable dish, "sayur lodeh". It comprises of cabbage, long beans, and carrots stewed in coconut milk with dried shrimp or fish for enhancing the taste. Depending on how much coconut milk is used, this dish could be either fattening or non-fattening. This particular food stall in Novena Square used a lot of thick coconut milk. It was no wonder that I felt it on my waist almost instantly! This was also the time when I did not exercise regularly. The bottom line was, I wasn't eating by my own rules or doing those things I knew I should be doing. What I can tell you is that the attitude I had at that time was one of carelessness and over-optimism, with the hope of getting away with it rather than taking the path of extreme caution and self-discipline. Why? I guess I just wanted a break. After all, I was just being human. I just wanted to taste the good food my colleagues were having. I didn't think it would hurt. But hurt it did because losing weight was always more difficult and it takes a much longer time than gaining it! As for the chocolates, I had them almost every day, be it Kit Kat, Cadbury Fun Pack, or Belgian — you name it! In retrospect, there was no permanent damage. But given the same scenario again, I would not deviate. It would be too risky. What if, for some reason(s), I could not lose my weight back? Once in a lifetime would be enough. Sticking to my plans would be safer and more rewarding.

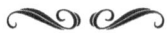

My Road of No Return
(2003 to Present)

11

My Road of No Return (2003 to Present)

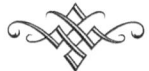

GIFAM

In 2003, I pursued a Bachelor of Science course in Holistic Nutrition from the Global Institute For Alternative Medicine (GIFAM). This course changed my life, in more than one respect. The principles on sugar, microwaving, pesticides, antibiotics, weight loss, hormones, artificial additives, potassium, exercise, and walking 4200 steps were just some of the new knowledge I gained.

Sugar Sabotaged My Weight

The first new piece of learning I put into practice was to give up candies, which had been part of my life for over ten years. Ask anyone in my family and they will tell you so. But in just one split moment, I decided to give it up when I realized to what dangers I was subjecting my body.[20] No more sleepiness, no more fear of low immunity for me. Sugar also causes the cross-linkage of collagen and elastin fibers in our skin, which leads to aging. It was following this truth that gave me the blessing of good health. Of course, it took longer to get rid of the supply of candies I had stored in my house before I came upon this knowledge. When they expired, I had no choice but to throw them away!

Canned Food

Another item I gave up was canned food, after learning it was full of preservatives, salt, sugar, and nitrites that were not only weight-gaining (because they caused our liver to work harder and have less energy to deal with fats and oils) but may also be carcinogenic in the long term. Occasionally, I would have luncheon meat, but that was about all. NO more canned sardines, canned tuna, canned corn, canned soup, or canned whatever.

MY ROAD OF NO RETURN (2003 TO PRESENT)

Discovering Potassium in 2003

There was a book in the GIFAM course by Dr Lynn Tan[21], which introduced the importance of detoxification for optimal health, including weight loss. One of the nutrients highlighted was potassium. Dr Lynn recommended a teaspoonful a day. So in that year, on the month of June, after a bout of indulgence and not being able to get below 85 pounds, I did take one teaspoon of potassium powder a day, and lost weight from 87 to 82 pounds in five straight days without changing my food intake or activity level. One caveat though, if you want to follow this: It only worked because at that time, my body was deficient in potassium. So how does one know if potassium will fix the stubborn weight plateau? I hate to break your heart, but there is no way of telling. (Or rather, no way that I know. But if you do, please let me know.) You just have to use it!! If it works, it works. The important lesson is to always be on the lookout for new ways, new information, and new tricks!

My latest discovery was that adding raw shredded garlic to my cabbage leads to satisfaction, which in turn helps me to feel satisfied on a smaller serving. It is magical. Another trick I used recently was to take two to three oil of oregano capsules (which smells exactly like the oregano spice used in pasta and pizzas) so that when I burped, I had a feeling of satiety. If my burp had oil of oregano in it, that meant there was still food in my tummy — and it was not yet time to eat. I won't recommend you follow this if you totally despise the flavor, taste, and smell of oregano. It can be an acquired taste.

The Importance of Sleep

I realized that when my mind was refreshed, I tended not to have food cravings. But when I didn't sleep well and suffered from brain fog, I developed food cravings that drove me to eat even though I was not hungry. This was probably because though I was not fully awake, I was expected to perform on the job, so eating meals, including snacks and drinking coffee with its thermic effect did something to jolt my circulation and give me temporary alertness. But the gain in weight as a result was too high a price to pay. So, as far as possible, for the latter part of my life, I would ensure that I slept well by not partaking in any taboo activities before sleep. The following I have identified to interfere with falling asleep smoothly:

- Eating sugary meals just before bedtime.

- Checking and sending emails at night.
- Surfing the internet (which is full of new information that causes excitement for a "want to know all" like me) before bedtime.
- Watching exciting movies or drama serials on TV.

The following are helpful to promote sleep (for me at least):

- Eating a light meal at least one hour before bedtime, and not consuming anything stimulating like coffee or cocoa drinks.
- Reading the newspaper or self-improvement books.
- Listening to a low-key presentation on tape.
- Just switching on the sound of my favorite movies and letting it roll till I fall asleep.
- Listening to Deepak Chopra, who has an extremely soothing voice, while I am falling asleep.
- Or simply breathe deeply and slowly in and out.
- Or just tell your mind: Be Silent!

Besides enabling me to feel refreshed and

strapped with willpower the following day, sleep also promoted my fat burning. When I get up in the morning, my body is usually hot like a furnace and my tummy relatively flatter than the night before. From here, I concluded that I must have burnt fat while I slept. This theory of mine has now been corroborated by experts in the field of anti-aging, weight loss, and fitness that I came across from various sources.[22]

My experience with this started only in my most recent years, well, after the year 2000 at least. Before this year, I had no consciousness of this phenomenon. I consider this a reprieve for me because I work so hard to fight off fat! It seems that my body goes into this fat burning phase some time after I fall asleep, which is around the time that **human growth hormone** (which helps burn fat and repair our worn-out cells) is released. Why I did not notice or experience this in my earlier years is again a mystery. It could be that due to better nutrient supplementation and eating the right foods, my physiology became optimal, and my metabolism was changing from one that was ultra slow to one that was more efficient. Or it could be that I was influenced by what I read in health magazines and books so much so that

MY ROAD OF NO RETURN (2003 TO PRESENT)

I manifested the idea into a physical fact. Not knowing the reason did not stop me from enjoying my newfound efficiency in burning fat. Tied in with this night-time fat burning was a higher resting body temperature. In other words, I could withstand cold temperatures but couldn't suffer hot temperatures. The only time I needed to wear a sweater would be in the cinema or a function room with temperatures tuned to below 22°C. So in case anyone has any qualms about sleeping, don't! Because it really helps burn fat!

Cortisol – The Stress Hormone

Often times in my years of weight management discovery, I had been licked by stress, in that when I was overwhelmed, I felt helpless and gave in to eating for comfort. My stress would come in all shapes and sizes. For example, if I had bloating due to IBS, the discomfort would give me a sense of annoyance and irritation that made me lose my judgement and self-control. Or, when I had to finish an essay or type a letter, I would go into negative stress, with knots in my stomach, which mimics hunger. As a result, times of negative stress were not welcome, as my natural tendency would be to reach out for food and gain weight. I hated that I could not master myself. Then one fine day, as I was routinely reading Let's Live magazine, I realized I was not alone. I read that our body produces a hormone called cortisol when we are under stress, and in most people this would cause an increase in eating urges as well as a tendency to put on weight around the middle. All this information was in tandem with my personal experiences. Knowing of this human condition spurred me on to develop counter tactics to eating. Self-talk and activities were my greatest strategies for overcoming it. I was successful only because I was determined and believed there was a way out!

On the contrary, positive stress, when doing something I like, even if within a limited time, caused me to expend more calories and slim down. Therefore, stress cuts both ways depending on how we perceive and respond to it. This could occur at a subconscious level.

Fasted on Days Off or Ate Less

This follows from the above in that on my days off, because there was no stress from work, my appetite would totally switch off. I welcomed this and took the chance to fast. Whether the fast was successful or not depended on how much I had deviated from my planned agenda the days before. The lesson I learned from this is that prevention is better than damage control. Other benefits of fasting are increased motivation and determination to succeed, mental alertness, emotional and physical well-being, body consciousness, plus sharpened senses, including the taste buds!

I Trusted What I Read (Past Tense)

Knowledge is empowering to me because I put into practice what I learn right away. But nothing less of conviction of course! Yet how many people read the same stuff I did but didn't come off with the same conviction. I should consider myself lucky to be able to trust whole-heartedly (take by faith) those who have done the research on our behalf. Not every piece of information on weight management and health would square with my experience, but then nothing does in life. So, I just do what I can and apply what I can. The result: I am better off than before!

I Ate by Numbers – A Calorie is a Calorie

For many years, I had cheated by eating more than I should every once in a while. Guilt did not kill, but not having a perfect body did! PLUS not being able to fit into my clothes! In a way, I was sabotaging myself. It was not until the year 2000 onwards that I finally bowed to the fact that a calorie is a calorie. The laws of cause and effect are immutable. What goes up must come down. What we eat must be used up or excreted. Otherwise, it gets stored as fat or causes disease. A man reaps what he sows. Period. What consequence did this realization have for me? Very simply: Do not cheat. Do not get away with it. Do not justify my overeating. Recognizing my self-deceitfulness empowered me to develop counter strategies to avoid overeating. It then became a pleasure to be precise. The reward: A shapely me.

Continued to be Nitpicky About Food

Since eating was so precious, I had to choose carefully. This was by no means easy, especially during times when I was overworked. So I developed a system of bringing food to work. The food was to be a precise amount (fist-sized) of boiled vegetables with one piece of minced meat or equivalent, and usually just a little or no carbohydrate, because I get these from snacks like buns and cakes and beverages. When someone offered me food, I would politely refuse. If the food offered was healthy, I would eat it in substitution of and not in addition to whatever I had prepared.

The Value of Spice

One thing I did right was to love having chilli, curries, and spices in my food. Although in my earlier years I did not know, chilli and turmeric found in curry powder does increase metabolic rate[23] by up to 25%. That is astounding, considering I did not have to increase my activity level.

Shopping for Clothes

Shopping for clothes burns calories and keeps the appetite down more than any other activity I partake in. When I shop for clothes, my entire being is engaged in decision-making, artistic appreciation, and creative thinking. That kind of shuts down every inclination to eat. Moreover, flitting from display to display, picking dress after dress and taking off and putting them on, and then taking them off again is physical activity that requires energy. Furthermore, moving from shop to shop also requires movement of the leg muscles and the state of urgency and positive energy I possess when shopping adds burning power to it all!

TV or Food, Not Both

During the time that Korean TV drama serials became popular in Singapore, I developed the unfortunate habit of eating while watching TV. I ate snack foods of all sorts — chocolate cookies, peanuts, salted crackers, and potato chips. I felt powerless at that time because a habit once formed is hard to break. During commercial breaks and when the movie got exciting or boring, I would reach for my snacks. So any which way, I was doomed. What made me finally change? Let's just say, my time had come, my eyes were opened, the scales fell from my eyes, and the veil was lifted. I saw my situation as it was. What did I see? A vicious cycle of making effort to slim down, finally slimming down, watching TV, then putting on weight again, turning my effort to naught, and then making the effort again, slimming down, and no sooner had I achieved this, fell into the old habit again with alarming though not unpredictable end results. All this fruitless energy was causing me to feel guilty and I wondered if one day I might never recover. So should I not stretch my chances too far? What if I gained weight and couldn't lose it again? In one split second, I made a decision to keep food and TV separate. After I made that declaration, I never went back to it. Our tongue has the power of life and death.

Dared to Eat Different

The world is unkind to people who are different. Some common labels are freaks and weirdoes. The same goes for people who have a low metabolism — because it shows in their weight if they are not careful. See, people who are obese are not necessarily those who eat the most or eat sinfully. Life was never fair from the beginning, so we should not expect it to be now. What we can do, however, is to accept ourselves, discover ourselves, and give ourselves what we need to have the best body. And that includes eating just the right amount of food for our low metabolism[24], nothing more, nothing less. The number of calories we need to stay alive is commensurate with our target weight. The heavier weights and those with higher metabolic rates would need more and therefore can enjoy eating more. The lower weights and those with lower metabolism who love food would just have to be content with eating less. Even though it seems we are in the minority, this has not been statistically confirmed. In order to fit in, I may just bow in to pressure to eat like the more privileged (those with higher metabolic rates). But I chose not to because the consequence would be gaining weight. Staying the same weight meant more to me as I would then remain confident and at ease with myself. So it followed that I had to look out for myself all the time when ordering food. Considering the ridicule I experienced when I was fat during my younger days, doing this was not difficult at all, even though it took effort and some persuasion to get food servers to give me exactly what I requested for. And this, despite the odd looks I got from them.

How did I place my order then? Well, a typical economical rice meal would be two tablespoonfuls of rice, a moderate amount of curry sauce (which has the herb turmeric, a metabolic enhancer), a serving of tofu, and a serving of pulpy vegetables, for example: broccoli and cabbage.

MY ROAD OF NO RETURN (2003 TO PRESENT)

Continued to Eat Everything with Vegetables

I ate everything with vegetables, and I mean everything that would be considered a serving of protein or a serving of carbohydrate. The only exceptions were chocolates, cakes, and bread (which I ate only occasionally and not every single day). Bread, I limit more than chocolates because of its high glycemic index[25], meaning it is absorbed quickly into the bloodstream and causes our blood sugar to rise. Once in a while, I eat food prepared by other people. Even so, I will always request for vegetables. If they were cooked in a way that was too oily, I would give it a miss.

I learned that if I ate food with vegetables, some of the fats and oils will get entangled in the fiber mass and get prevented from being absorbed. So that has been my eating habit for a long time. Fiber from vegetables also prevents constipation, which is conducive to weight loss.

If I deviated from this, I made it the exception and NOT the Rule.

I found my way back through trial and error. I was not intransigent.

HOW I LOST TWENTY POUNDS...

My Fist-Sized Meals

From 1989 onwards, I had been eating fist-sized meals by intuition without calling it such. I used to tell people my meal size was like that of a "char siew pau" (a Chinese steamed meat bun) simply because it felt comfortable eating that amount, which I found neither too filling nor depriving. Later, the term progressed to "8 oz meals", and finally, after reading Shawn Philips "ABsolution" in 2004, I started using the term "fist-sized". Anyway, this sounded more refined. I was overjoyed that I finally found someone who was more disciplined about food than I was. Moreover, he is a renowned nutritional scientist and resistance training guru ("abs" to be specific). I felt I was part of a community of enlightened beings. If you read about his lifestyle, you will find that he is far more strict than I in terms of eating habits. Eating just the right amount and not more was essential to his success formula. It's the same for me. Caveat: In his book, Mr Phillips recommended fist-sized for each of the portions of vegetables, protein, and carbohydrate, whereas for myself it was fist-sized for all three COMBINED, plus a little more. Only recently, in 2006, did I realize I could eat a little more and found myself closer to following the recommended fist-sized for each of the food types. Even so, I seldom finished every single morsel.

Continued to Observe Myself

"I am different today than the day before."

Like other people, my body changes over time and so do my food sensitivities and preferences. (It is thought that our food preferences may reflect our nutrient needs.) This could have something to do with the circumstances and challenges we face each day, which utilize or deplete nutrients from our bodies as we live and function. Collateral to this is the fact that my appetite changes from day to day (though not by a far margin). So I pay attention to this, adjust accordingly, and do not insist on eating the same food or same serving size every day. However, they are not far off from the fist-sized portions I was talking about earlier and never more than one and a half times.

So how did I know when to change food (menu) or when it was permissible to eat a little more? Well, it is very much more intuition than perfect science. When I get "sick" of a certain food, it is high time to change. Otherwise, I would be sabotaging myself as I would then feel that I have not enjoyed my meal, feel deprived, and allow food cravings to creep in. This could easily trigger off an unwanted binge! Secondly, I knew I could eat a little more when my activities for a particular day expended more calories than usual. For example, if instead of watching movies and reading, I decided to clean house on my day off, that would entitle me to perhaps, an extra snack or two for that day and FOR THAT DAY ONLY. In other words, by listening to my body and going with my metabolic flow, I avoided eating more than I should. This way, not only did I enjoy eating, but successfully maintained my weight as well.

Prepared for Temptation

"Desire is crouching at the door but we must master it!"[26]

This is so true of food, especially for someone like me who loves to eat. I believe the majority of my fellow humans share the same love. The thing is: I have decided not to give in to it. Temporary pleasure I can stomach (or rather enjoy), but NOT the longer-term pain of sluggishness, depression, low metabolism, and loss of self-confidence. Because mental clarity and emotional well-being were of utmost importance to me, I was strict with myself and constantly reminded myself that breaking the rules was simply NOT worth it! If through carelessness, I did slip up, how fast I recovered from my setback in weight depended on how fortunate I was in finding the right activities to participate in. For example, being involved in a three-day seminar or a boot camp would mean pretty much eating only at the allotted time slots. That meant fewer calories consumed. In addition to this, networking with others usually causes a drop in appetite. Why? Because conversation is such a filler! As it is written, *"From the fruit of his mouth, a man's stomach is filled, with the harvest from his lips he is satisfied."* (Proverbs 18:20) Since these activities are few and far between and costs money to attend, it would be better in the first place, not to succumb to any temptation. Besides, losing weight usually takes double, if not more, of the time than gaining it. Just not my thing!

"Power of One"

Occasionally, I slipped into the habit of eating sweets and chocolates for dessert and found my weight creeping up by about half a pound a day.

When that happened, I had to put a stop to it. I did this using the above mantra, which simply means that "if you have to eat it, eat only one"! To my delight, it worked amazingly well. Now, to me that was powerful and effective.

Self-Talk

This was my most important and successful weight maintenance strategy. I constantly reminded myself about the consequences of being overweight — that I was different in my metabolism, that I couldn't join others in their festive eating much as I wanted to. I had to accept myself the way I was, including how many calories I could burn. Examples of some of my self-talk are (and applied only when eating was inappropriate):

- "Stop feeding yourself, you skinny ass!"
- "Better to let it go to waste than go to your waist."
- "If you want to overeat, wait till tomorrow."
- "When I am slim, I can wear anything, go anywhere, date anyone."
- "No time is a good time to eat." (Applied only when eating was inappropriate.)

MY ROAD OF NO RETURN (2003 TO PRESENT)

- "Eating is not an option."
- "Sorry, I am sculpting my body."
- "Eat as though not eating." (*This was influenced by the Apostle Paul's philosophy of detachment as espoused in 1 Corinthians 7:29-31.*)
- "When you're are at home, you are not." (Given that the likelihood of "letting go" on food would be at home rather than when at work or a social function.)
- "When in doubt, err on the side of under eating."
- "Fat is slow dying."
- "Count till 3000!"

I would like to elaborate on the third one ("If you want to overeat, wait till tomorrow"), which is my favorite. When I was tempted to overeat, I would tell myself to wait till tomorrow. When tomorrow came, I told myself exactly the same thing, and yet again the next day. That way, I would end up never overeating! Wonderful! Looking back, I feel that I have grown out of saying this because it has become part of my subconscious — a habit, if you like. In other words, not overeating became effortless.

"Counting till 3000" was really fun for me. I

noticed that whenever I counted till 200, I would totally lose any desire to eat, as by that time, I would have found something useful or absorbing to do.

Ate Only When Hungry

The mistake I sometimes made was to eat the minute I felt hungry. Sometimes it paid to wait a little longer to confirm that I was experiencing true hunger and not some food craving caused by stress or malnutrition or even thirst or dehydration. For example, if I drank a cup of tea or coffee first thing in the morning in response to a hungry feeling or what I thought was a hungry feeling, and the feeling of hunger goes away, that meant what I needed in the first place was fluids rather than solid food. In fact, the tea or coffee would fill me up to the extent that I sometimes did not have to eat till noon.

Love – The Panacea

The Bible constantly reminds us to live a life of love. Incidentally, having this emotion does good for weight control. One way I apply this is to literally watch romantic movies, which generates feelings of warmth and healing. Also, in line with this is loving my life, my work, my routines, and activities. Make less the transgressions of others. Forgive. The result of living a life of love is lowered appetite, lowered food cravings, lowered snacking (food transgressions), and great emotional well-being, which ultimately led to physical well-being! What goes around comes around.

Chromium Picolinate (Jan 2004)

After eating too many chocolates during Christmas of 2003, I could not get my weight below 85 again. But I decided to give chromium picolinate a shot because I had been reading about this supplement for more than five years and had never put it to the test. Within three days of 400mcg of chromium picolinate per day, I was back to my usual 85 pounds. So what does chromium do? Well:

- **Chromium** spares muscle and muscle burns more fat.
- It raises our metabolic rate and enables us to burn more calories per unit time.
- It makes our cells more responsive to insulin. As a result, glucose molecules get utilized rather than remain in our blood

stream to be converted to fat eventually.
- Chromium reduces food and sugar cravings.

Why, after working in a health store or stores for more than ten years, have I not used this? Again, my answer is: I do not know. It may have something to do with timing again, which meant that I would be led to do a thing only when it was right for me.

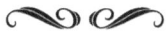

What After All
Is Ideal Weight?

12

What After All Is Ideal Weight?

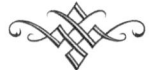

This has been the most difficult part of my book. What I am saying here is not instructional, just some food for thought. Your ideal weight is what you will be most comfortable with, the most ravishing, most attractive you. Of course, this weight may change over time, a pound off here and half a pound on there, but nothing too extreme and which will still allow you to look your greatest. Look around you and observe the different body types you see. Nobody is the same. There is no similar body shape, just similar body types! And stop comparing yourself with others. We were meant to be different. The bottom line is you have to make up your mind what weight you want to be. I had to make up my mind once upon a time. At 80 pounds, I was waif thin, but there was no enjoyment of food. At 85 pounds, I looked sexier and could eat a little more. So whether 80 or 85, I would allow myself only to vary between these two weights. Beyond 85, I would just look mediocre and I would have to change dress sizes, which isn't very economical. As time moves on, perhaps my ideal weight may be a little different again. Recently, my weight has moved up a pound or two, but that could be the result of taking human growth hormone releasers, which probably contributed to a gain in muscle weight rather than fat weight. The important thing is that I have to be all right with the gain of a pound or two, which fortunately, I am.

And don't listen to others, whether family, friends or researchers. Your self-concept or image is more important. You have to live with your body, not they! With regard to researchers, William Herbert Sheldon has identified 88 body types, but summarized these to three for simplicity.[27] The point of this is that there are too many different body types to make any generalizations of what ideal weight is! This, coupled with the fact that the BMI (Body Mass Index), a way of estimating healthy weight by dividing a person's weight by the square of his height, is based on averages and not absolutes, means that to date, there is no perfect tool to help you determine what weight you ought to be. Don't trust these entirely. Trust yourself. Use your own judgement. Use the mirror, and use your clothes. How you feel about the way you look is ultimately more important. It is your weight to love, so BE the weight YOU want to be.

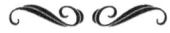

In Summary

13

In Summary

I lost 20 pounds and kept it off because:

- I learnt the caloric value of food.

- I was determined.

- I observed myself and developed awareness
  of my metabolic type, my food sensitivities,
  and food preferences.

- I kept my activity level up by engaging in
  walking as an exercise and chose a career
  that burned calories.

- I kept regular hours of sleep and work,
  exercise and eating, as best I could.

- I made vegetables a substantial part of
  every meal. I ate vegetables with other food
  so that not all the fats and oils would be
  absorbed and also because they shortened

elimination time.

- I avoided sweet desserts, soft drinks, and concentrated candies whenever possible. Also, I used sugar sparingly, and through the years, this gets less and less.

- If I had a sweet tooth (and this not always), I used "the power of one" for chocolates and candy.

- I learnt to manage stress. I learnt to deal with stress by not responding with eating but with some other activity, like dancing, running, or walking, which lowers the weight gaining hormone, cortisol, or simply engaged in self-talk or dived into some absorbing activity.

- I fasted occasionally.

- I ate spices that picked up metabolism (curries, chillies).

- I learnt to use oils sparingly and avoided deep-fried food, which is bad for my weight and skin. If I do eat them, it would be an exception not a habit.

- I erred on the side of under eating. And if I overate, that would be the exception, not habit.

- I never ate in response to other people's

invitations when my body tells me it is not time to eat.

- I used potassium and chromium picolinate supplements at one time or another.
- I dropped crackers, potato chips, and canned food from my diet, which slow the elimination process and are full of additives that are weight gaining. And also, I avoided, to the best of my ability, hidden salt in cereals and beverage creamers.
- I accumulated and created taglines, self-talk, slogans, and when I was tempted, used these to resist and overcome eating temptations.
- I accumulated knowledge from all over, read stories of other people's successes, and applied as much as I could to my own case. I practiced all I read and discovered.
- I engaged in activities that fanned my passion and energy.

I Had Setbacks Because:
- I did not practice what I knew.
- I gave in to temptation.
- I let up on my efforts because I was tired, and I was tired either because I did not

sleep well or because I was depressed about something.

How I Recovered from my Setbacks:

By any means possible:

- I ate less than three meals.
- I ate smaller meals (smaller than 8 oz at times).
- I ate obscenely little.
- I ate only vegetables.
- I ate further apart (six-seven hours).
- I dropped the candies and chocolates and tidbits high in salt.
- I dropped the starchy carbohydrates too.
- Strictly no cheating on the above.
- I walked longer than usual.
- I kept physically active.
- I involved myself in some passion.
- I went on a fast and stuck to the times my mind had fixed even though my body didn't want to follow. After a while my body would adjust. All I had to do was say No and keep saying No!

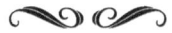

Pointers for Readers

14

Pointers for Readers

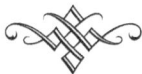

▪ Learn the calorie values of food. The calorie value of food is underrated. You may have someone who drank six cups of coffee that day and says she/he hasn't lost a single pound though she/he hasn't eaten anything for that day. The fact is, those six cups of coffee may have 600 calories depending on whether there is sugar and creamer in it. On the other hand, you may encounter someone who ate three pieces of pineapple and says she hasn't eaten anything. True, no rice, no bread, but those three slices of pineapple may have at least 200 calories in it.

▪ Having no appetite or low appetite is good for a weight loss incumbent, at least for a short spell of time. Some may disagree. I say so because this means your body is cleansed and well-nourished. Impaction of the colon or autointoxication will lead to cravings that will cause us to eat more.

▪ Be always vigilant for pitfalls, i.e. know your own weaknesses for food(s). They will always be with you, so the earlier you accept them, the sooner you are able to deal with them.

▪ Stick to your guns. Foods suitable for your friends and others may not be suitable for you and cause you to gain weight. Examples are cheese, butter, durians, and bananas. All of us are different metabolically.

▪ We will always eat more than we want. This is human nature. This is how we were tuned or programmed, like a survival trait. I do not know why. But we should just stop eating when three quarters full.

▪ An adjunct to **"stop when ¾ full"** is "stop when your body tells you to". This is even more powerful. The difference is that your body may tell you to stop even before the food is half finished for whatever reason. Under such circumstances, trust your body, obey it, and stop. Your obedience unlocks the keys to all the right memories and sets into motion a continuous string of right choices, but disobedience might interrupt the smooth path that was meant to be in the first place. Domino effect.

▪ Beware of social eaters. Join them for a drink, but avoid ordering anything even if for free, unless it is your proper mealtime and unless there is the type of food you can eat.

▪ Sleeping well and chasing away the blues are absolutely necessary for staying at the right weight unless you are the type to lose appetite when depressed. Most people tend to eat more when depressed.

▪ Listen to your body. This could mean your body will tell you whether you should eat a certain food now or later. For instance, the last time I ate an ice cream cone from McDonald's was last week, which meant that it could be a good six months later before I have my next. My creature of habit tells me I should eat one tonight too, but my body says: "No, wait a day or two." Come tomorrow, my body may say "wait a week or so". At every stage, your body is always right. Just make sure you are sensitized to it.

▪ How do we sensitize our bodies? Go on a cleansing program. Eat only vegetables. Begin to eat slimming foods: vegetables and low glycemic index carbohydrates. Decrease the salt, additives, and sugars.

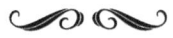

FAQs

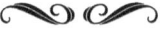

15

FAQs

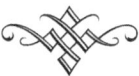

Q. *Doesn't seeing another eat a large amount cause you to do the same?*

A. No. I understand that my body is different than theirs. So they are entitled to eat whatever amount they want. I don't feel guilty or bad that I can't join them. Would you expect a deaf person to hear or a blind person to literally "see"? It's the same with metabolic types. You can't expect a slow burner to be a fast burner and vice versa.

Q. *Did you ever feel like letting go and just eat all you can?*

A. Of course. But then I would be inviting one of the things I shun most — being overweight, depressed, and out of shape. We can't cheat nature. There are always consequences when we deviate from the right path. Indeed, we reap what we sow. Anyway, I had my quota of little experiments to investigate what would become of me if I did just that. In 2003, I bought a packet of "char siew rice" (roast pork rice) and ate every single grain of it. After that, I was fat and sick for three days. How many rules did I break? Rule 1: Always eat your food with vegetables (fiber) Rule 2: Finish when three quarters full. Rule 3: For your metabolic rate, keep your carbohydrate intake low. (One packet of rice amounts to 600 calories. My usual was two tablespoons or 100 calories.)

Q. *What do you do during a ten-course Chinese dinner or at a buffet dinner celebration with relatives?*

A. During a ten-course Chinese dinner, I would avoid the deep-fried food and sweet desserts. I chit-chat in-between or visit the rest room. What I eat is mostly the sharks fin soup (three-quarters of it), the tomatoes, broccoli and cucumbers, a slice of roast chicken perhaps, and that's it. If steamed fish or tofu is served, I help myself to more. As for buffets, I fill up my plate abundantly with 70 percent slushy vegetables. Examples are cabbages, kuah, long beans or French beans, and broccoli.

The other 30 percent would be two tablespoons of rice plus whatever meat is in the offering. This could be tofu, minced meat, roast chicken or something stir-fried, plus plenty of curry sauce (if available) and sambal chilli sauce (if available). Mostly, I will finish the vegetables and leave some of the rest.

Q. *Would you agree with some critiques that by going on a permanent low calorie diet, we would be undernourished with the RDAs of essential nutrients?*
A. NO. In fact I would say that we would be malnourished even on, say, a 2000 calorie-a-day diet because the density of nutrients in food today just isn't what it used to be 50 years ago due to over farming and food processing. The solution would be to pick more fresh foods and take a multivitamin formula plus essential oil supplement to ensure we have a guaranteed RDI of nutrients to function (optimally) on.

Q. *Were there other times you were called fat?*
A. Most certainly. I remember being called so by my church mate, a stranger, an associate, and a colleague. That makes four. And there are probably

other instances by other people I have not recalled. All of them meant well and I have them to thank, because without their honest feedback, I would not be where I am today.

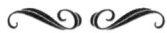

A Final Word

A Final Word

There you have it!

I hope this story of mine has left you feeling motivated, inspired, and encouraged in your fight against being overweight. For those of you high metabolic types who do not share the same weight challenges, I hope you have found my story entertaining. At least, it helps you understand those who suffer from weight challenges a little better.

If there is anything I have written that you would like to ask me more about, please email me at How_I_Lost@yahoo.com. (with underscore: How_I_Lost). It would be my pleasure and honor to answer you.

Thank you and once again,

Happy weight maintenance!

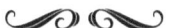

Footnotes

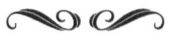

Footnotes

1. It has been discovered that the human body needs two essential fatty acids called omega 3 and omega 6, and these are rather scant in our modern diets. Source: Udo Erasmus "Fats that Heal, Fats that Kill". However, this misperception did not do me any harm because most of the oils in cooked food were bad oils anyway, according to Dr Udo.

2. Carbohydrates become sugars upon digestion. Excess sugar molecules join together to form fats.

3. This is alternating diarrhea and constipation, plus bloating and occasional stomach cramping. An excellent e-book on Irritable Bowel Syndrome would be "The IBS Cure" by Rachit Dayal, 2007

4. These were found in fried kway teow, fried carrot cake, hokkien mee, and ice kachang, just to name a few. Anything that is ground rather

than whole is refined. Their surface area is larger, so they get absorbed faster and cause a rise in insulin levels, which leads to fat storage.

5. For anyone interested to know how misinformed we are today about fats and oils, I would recommend Udo Erasmus "Fats that Heal, Fats that Kill".

6. At that time, I was eating three moderately sized meals a day and sleeping seven hours.

7. To make ends meet, I ate really cheap food, luncheon meat, and crinkle fries, which (you probably wouldn't have guessed if I didn't tell) was deep-fried! At that time, I really, really didn't know about the harmful effects of deep-frying. Dr Udo's book was first published in 1993!

8. From the Aug 1998 issue of Let's Live magazine (a US publication).

9. A sweet dessert of shredded ice piled atop cooked red beans (from whence the word "kachang" comes, which means "bean" in Malay), artificially flavored, pink and green agar cubes and a few palm seeds (atap chee). The mountain of shredded ice is drizzled with artificially flavored colored syrup, a little evaporated milk, and garnished with

a tablespoon of canned sweet corn. This is commonly served in Singapore and Malaysia.

10. By Martin Katahn, PhD

11. By Fred A. Stutman, MD

12. Popiah - A vegetable wrap consisting of a thin, wheat flour pancake skin filled with stewed turnip (the most abundant item in the filling, which is stir fried and stewed with soy sauce, a little shrimp, and shredded carrot for flavor), some bean sprouts, a piece of lettuce, a little fried shredded batter, a little ground roasted peanuts, a tablespoon or two of mashed hard boiled egg (or shredded omelet). The popiah skin is first spread with a little chilli sauce, sweet sauce, and garlic paste before wrapping the filling. This is a common dish in Singapore and Malaysia.

13. One example is Shawn Phillips "ABsolution" wherein Mr Phillips described the fist-sized meal and advocates sticking to pre-planned amounts of food so that we would get hungry only at the right intervals. The difference between his fist-sized portions and mine were that his proportions were fist-sized **each** for **carbohydrate, protein, and vegetables** whereas mine was **fist-sized for all three** most

of the time!

14. I cannot remember the title of his book. All I remember is that he was a fruitarian and was very brave and radical, as he experimented with his own body as to what foods were good and which were bad for the health.

15. Available now online at www.bragg.com

16. There are no more copies of this for distribution. However, one may log on to www.hpb.gov.sg to access the web-based food composition table, "Food Info Search" on the HPB Homepage.

17. I have a Bachelor of Science degree in Holistic Nutrition from GIFAM (The Global Institute For Alternative Medicine)

18. For those unfamiliar with this, chendol is an Asian cold dessert with gula melaka (palm sugar) and coconut milk (the main fluid ingredients), as well as cooked red beans, green stuff, and seaweed jelly (or agar) as the solid ingredients. The best way to find out is just to go to your nearest food court when you visit Singapore or Malaysia and ask for it. It's simply delightful, if not for the aftermath.

19. A US publication, Aug 1998 issue

20. Among other things, sugar feeds bacteria, yeast and cancer cells, and accelerates aging

by inducing cross-linkages in collagen. It also brings about blood sugar imbalances when taken in excess.

21. Dr Lynn Tan (ND), "You can Regain Youth and Health through Detoxification and Rejuvenation".

22. One article I found was on the American National Sleep Foundation website. It says: "Sleep helps us thrive by contributing to a healthy immune system, and can also balance our appetites by helping to regulate levels of the hormones **ghrelin** and **leptin**, which play a role in our feelings of hunger and fullness. **So when we're sleep deprived, we may feel the need to eat more, which can lead to weight gain.**" Another source is a blog post entitled, "Burn Fat While You Sleep" on 21 Mar 2006 by Joe DiAngelo, a coveted fitness expert and personal trainer in New York City, on his website musclebomb.com. On this page he says: "If you sleep less than seven hours per night, you'll block the production of **human growth hormone** that will cause you to gain weight. If you don't get enough sleep, leptin levels will go down and you will feel more hungry the next day."

23. Deepak Chopra "Magical Mind, Magical Body".
24. It is hoped that metabolism can be increased with proper nutrition and metabolic enhancers such as chromium picolinate, guarana herb, CLA (Conjugated Linoleic Acid) and L-carnitine, but since the degree of improvement is tough to determine and is not measurable to a specific degree, it would be best to err on the side of caution and eat according to one's estimated metabolism especially if it is a low one.
25. Glycemic Index (GI). This is a numeric measure of how fast a carbohydrate is broken down into its simple sugar unit and enters the bloodstream. The lower the GI, the better.
26. My adaptation of Genesis 4:7
27. "The Men's Health Hard-Body Plan" by Larry Keller

www.ingramcontent.com/pod-product-compliance
Lightning Source LLC
Chambersburg PA
CBHW061259280526
45784CB00002B/823